ULTIMATE ILEOSTOMY DIET HANDBOOK

Eating Well, Living Well

The Culinary Strategies For A Life Filled With Flavor And Vitality

DR. SOFIA SILAS

Table of Contents

CHAPTER ONE

Introduction

Living with an ileostomy may bring several obstacles, notably in terms of optimal nutrition and food. An ileostomy is a surgical treatment that diverts a section of the small intestine to a hole in the abdominal wall, enabling waste to skip the colon.

This change in the digestive tract may have a substantial influence on nutrient absorption and digestion, demanding careful dietary and nutritional considerations to maintain general health and wellness.

Understanding Ileostomy

An ileostomy is often used to treat a variety of medical disorders, including inflammatory bowel disease, colorectal cancer, and familial polyposis. During the surgery, the physician inserts a stoma—a surgically formed opening—in the abdominal wall through which waste products stream into an external pouch.

This rerouting of the digestive system avoids the colon, causing alterations in bowel habits and nutritional absorption.

Benefits Of Specialized Diets

Following ileostomy surgery, a tailored diet may provide various advantages to those transitioning to life with an ostomy. A well-planned diet may help control symptoms including diarrhea, dehydration, and electrolyte imbalances, which are significant concerns for ileostomies.

A customized diet may also improve food absorption, enhance digestive health, and lower the risk of issues like blockages or discomfort at the stoma site.

Nutritional Needs After Ileostomy Surgery

Individuals who have had ileostomy surgery may notice changes in their dietary needs as a result of changes in digestive function. The lack of the colon, which is essential for water and electrolyte absorption, might result in greater fluid and electrolyte loss via the stoma.

As a result, maintaining proper hydration and electrolyte balance is critical for avoiding dehydration and associated problems.

Furthermore, those with ileostomies may have a lower absorption of some nutrients, including vitamin B12, fat-soluble vitamins (A, D, E, and K), and electrolytes like salt and potassium.

As a result, it is essential to include nutrient-dense foods in the diet and, in certain situations, supplement with vitamins or minerals to avoid deficiencies.

CHAPTER TWO

Navigating Digestive Changes

It may be difficult to adjust to the digestive changes caused by an ileostomy, especially in the first few days after surgery. Many people have more frequent bowel movements, looser stools, and changes in stool consistency, which may influence their nutrition and meal planning.

Working collaboratively with healthcare specialists, such as dietitians or ostomy nurses, is critical to addressing these changes and developing appropriate symptom management measures.

Developing A Healthy Eating Plan

Developing a healthy eating plan after ileostomy surgery entails choosing foods that promote optimum digestion, alleviate symptoms, and offer necessary nutrients. Here are some basic dietary advice for people with ileostomies:

1. Choose readily digested meals, such as prepared vegetables, lean meats, and delicate fruits.

2. Introduce fiber gradually to avoid digestive difficulties

including gas, bloating, and blockages. Concentrate on soluble fibers found in oats, barley, and fruits, as opposed to insoluble fibers found in bran or raw vegetables.

3. Stay hydrated by consuming lots of fluids, including water and electrolyte-rich beverages such as sports drinks or coconut water. Limiting coffee and alcohol intake might also assist in avoiding dehydration.

4. Balance macronutrients: Eat a variety of carbs, proteins, and fats to maintain energy and promote general health. To achieve

adequate nutrition, choose lean proteins, healthy fats, and complex carbs.

5. Portion control: Eating smaller, more frequent meals throughout the day might alleviate symptoms like diarrhea and enhance nutritional absorption. Focus on portion management and pay attention to your body's hunger and fullness signals.

Individuals with ileostomies may design a healthy eating plan that meets their nutritional requirements while also improving their quality of life by adhering to these dietary recommendations and working closely with healthcare providers. Regular monitoring and modifications may be required as digestive function stabilizes and dietary tolerances develop over time.

Individuals living with an ileostomy must maintain good nutrition and dietary habits to promote their general health and well-being. Individuals may negotiate digestive changes, manage symptoms efficiently, and construct a healthy eating plan customized to their requirements by knowing the unique obstacles associated with an ileostomy, implementing a specialized diet, and working closely with healthcare specialists. Individuals with ileostomies may live full lives and have a higher quality of life after surgery provided they get sufficient nutrition and assistance.

Techniques For Ileostomy-Simple Meal Planning, And Snack Ideas For Sustained Energy

A balanced plate is more than simply filling it with food; it also includes a range of tasty components, proper cooking methods, meal planning, and snacks for sustained energy. Understanding these components is critical whether you're dealing with special dietary demands, such as those necessary for an ileostomy, or just seeking general health and well-being.

Exploring Flavored Ingredients: Flavor is the foundation for pleasurable meals. Incorporating a variety of components not only improves flavor but also provides nutritional balance. Vegetables such as spinach, bell peppers, and broccoli provide brilliant colors and critical vitamins to your menu. Fruits like berries, oranges, and apples are naturally sweet and contain antioxidants. Whole grains such as quinoa, brown rice, and oats include fiber and complex carbs, which give long-lasting energy.

Lean proteins, such as chicken, fish, tofu, and beans, include important amino acids required for muscle repair and general health. Don't forget about healthy fats like avocados, almonds, and olive oil, which promote satiety and support essential biological activities.

Cooking Tips For Ileostomy-Friendly Meals

Cooking for those who have an ileostomy takes great care to prevent causing pain or consequences. It is important to use cooking techniques that promote easy digestion.

 Steaming, baking, grilling, and poaching are gentle methods for preserving the nutritional value of foods without adding additional fat or creating discomfort.

Avoiding too spicy or strongly seasoned foods might assist in minimizing intestinal upset. Furthermore, ensuring that vegetables and fruits are completely cooked and digested may help digestion and reduce the chance of blockages.

Meal Planning Made Simple: Meal planning is an essential part of keeping a healthy diet, particularly for those who have unique dietary needs. Begin by planning a weekly meal with a range of nutrients and tastes.

Include items from all dietary categories to maintain a well-balanced diet. Take stock of cupboard supplies and plan meals around what you currently have to reduce waste and save money. Preparing meals ahead of time may help to simplify hectic weeknights and limit the temptation to eat less healthful quick items.

CHAPTER THREE

Snack Ideas For Sustained Energy

Snacks are essential for sustaining energy levels throughout the day, particularly for people with unique dietary demands. Choose snacks that include protein, carbs, and healthy fats to give a balanced supply of energy. Greek yogurt and berries, whole grain crackers with hummus, and apple slices with almond butter are some examples. Nuts and seeds are convenient and nutrient-dense snacks that can be consumed alone or combined with homemade trail mix.

Fresh fruits and vegetables with a small amount of cheese or nut butter make for a tasty and nutritious combination. Aim for snacks that are portable and simple to prepare, allowing you to refuel whenever hunger strikes without sacrificing nutrition.

To summarize, creating a balanced plate entails more than just deciding what to eat; it also entails selecting flavorful ingredients, using appropriate cooking techniques, planning meals effectively, and incorporating snacks for sustained energy.

Individuals can enjoy delicious and nourishing meals that support overall health and well-being by experimenting with different ingredients, using gentle cooking methods, practicing efficient meal planning, and choosing nutritious snacks, whether they are managing specific dietary needs or simply seeking optimal nutrition.

A holistic approach to nutrition and well-being includes hydration strategies for optimal health, mindful eating practices, dietary adaptations, managing digestive symptoms, addressing common concerns, and dining out with confidence.

In today's fast-paced world, where convenience frequently trumps health, it is critical to pay attention to these aspects of dietary habits to live a balanced and nourishing lifestyle.

Hydration Tips For Optimal Health

Water is the essence of life, and staying hydrated is critical for overall health and bodily function. Hydration requirements differ from person to person, influenced by age, weight, activity level, and climate.

A general guideline is to consume at least eight glasses of water per day, but individual needs may vary. Monitoring urine color can be an easy way to determine hydration levels; pale yellow urine indicates adequate hydration, whereas dark yellow or amber urine may indicate dehydration. Additionally, incorporating hydrating foods such as fruits and vegetables into meals can help with overall fluid intake.

Mindful eating involves being present and aware of the entire eating experience, including flavors, textures, and bodily sensations. This practice encourages slowing down during meals, savoring each bite, and paying attention to hunger and fullness cues.

By practicing mindful eating, individuals can cultivate a healthier relationship with food, reduce overeating, and improve digestion. Techniques such as chewing food thoroughly, eating without distractions, and recognizing emotional triggers for eating can support mindful eating habits.

Adapting Recipes For Dietary Needs

With the prevalence of food allergies, intolerances, and dietary preferences, it's essential to adapt recipes to accommodate various dietary needs.

This may involve substituting ingredients to avoid allergens, reducing sugar or salt content, or modifying cooking methods to align with specific dietary preferences, such as vegetarianism or veganism. Experimenting with alternative ingredients and exploring new cooking techniques can open up a world of culinary possibilities while ensuring that meals remain nutritious and satisfying for everyone.

Managing Digestive Symptoms

Digestive pain, such as bloating, gas, and indigestion, may substantially impair quality of life and general well-being. Managing digestive issues frequently entails identifying trigger foods and making dietary alterations appropriately.

Keeping a food journal may help monitor symptoms and uncover likely reasons. Additionally, consuming gut-friendly foods such as probiotics, fiber-rich fruits and vegetables, and fermented foods like yogurt and kimchi helps improve digestive health.

Consulting with a healthcare practitioner or certified dietitian may give more information on treating particular digestive concerns.

CHAPTER FOUR

Addressing Common Issues

Nutrition is a complicated and diverse component of health, and several common issues may emerge when it comes to dietary choices. These issues might vary from weight control and vitamin deficits to food safety and sustainability. Addressing these challenges involves a mix of education, awareness, and practical methods.

For example, concentrating on complete, nutrient-dense meals may help address dietary shortages, while exercising portion control and regular physical exercise are critical components of weight management. Staying knowledgeable about food safety requirements and supporting sustainable food practices may also help to general well-being.

Maintaining a healthy diet may be challenging while dining out. However, with the appropriate tactics, you can enjoy great meals with confidence. When eating out, it's a good idea to explore healthier selections or request menu adjustments to accommodate dietary restrictions.

Choosing grilled or steamed foods versus fried or highly sauced choices will help you consume fewer calories and fat. Furthermore, being attentive to portion sizes and exercising moderation may make eating out a more pleasurable and healthy experience.

To summarize, combining hydration measures, mindful eating habits, recipe adjustments, digestive symptom management, addressing common concerns, and dining out with confidence are all important components of maintaining a balanced and nutritious diet.

Individuals who prioritize these factors may improve their overall health and well-being by making educated decisions that are tailored to their own dietary requirements and tastes. With careful attention to these areas, obtaining maximum health via diet becomes not only possible but also pleasurable and sustainable in the long run.

Travel Tips For Ileostomy Patients

Traveling may be a rewarding experience, but people with ileostomies may face particular problems. However, with proper planning and preparation, it is possible to enjoy excursions and discover new locations with assurance. Here are some helpful hints for ileostomy sufferers to make their journeys easier and more pleasurable.

First and foremost, carry a enough amount of ostomy supplies. This comprises pouches, glue, skin barriers, wipes, and any other products required to change the ostomy equipment.

It's a good idea to pack extra materials than you think you'll need for the trip, just in case of unexpected situations or delays.

When packing, divide goods across many bags or baggage in case one is lost or forgotten. Furthermore, keeping a compact travel kit with emergency supplies in carry-on luggage enables easy access during flights or extended excursions.

Before going on a vacation, it is important to research the destination's amenities and accessibility. Identify nearby hospitals or medical institutions that can treat ostomy-related situations. Additionally, acquaint yourself with local pharmacies where ostomy supplies may be acquired if necessary.

Planning meals when traveling is critical for ileostomy sufferers. Choosing bland, easily digested meals may help avoid stomach problems and discomfort. It is recommended that you avoid items that might create blockages or gas accumulation, such as seeds, nuts, raw vegetables, and some fruits. It is also important to remain hydrated by drinking lots of water and avoiding excessive coffee and alcohol usage.

Maintaining a consistent eating schedule and tracking food intake may assist control of bowel motions and reduce the likelihood of leaks or accidents. Bringing snacks and portable, non-perishable foods may give handy alternatives for extended excursions or when access to appropriate meals is restricted.

When using public facilities, carrying a discreet pouch disposal bag or pouch deodorizer may help you retain your privacy and control stench. Using accessible facilities wherever feasible may also help to minimize the difficulties associated with changing an ostomy device in tight or filthy situations.

CHAPTER FIVE
Socializing And Celebrating With Food

Food is an important part of social events and celebrations, but it may be difficult for ileostomy patients to navigate these circumstances. However, with a good attitude and some practical measures, it is possible to enjoy holiday celebrations without jeopardizing health or comfort.

One way is to be forthright with hosts or event organizers about any food limitations or preferences linked to the ostomy. Offering to bring food that meets your dietary requirements guarantees there is at least one safe alternative available. Alternatively, eating ahead of time or bringing a modest snack might assist manage food-related worries during social occasions.

Staying Motivated Throughout Your Journey

Living with an ileostomy has its obstacles, but being motivated and optimistic is critical for general well-being. Setting realistic objectives and recognizing results, no matter how modest, may boost motivation and create a feeling of accomplishment.

Engaging in activities that offer pleasure and satisfaction, such as pursuing hobbies, spending time with loved ones, or discovering new interests, may help you keep a cheerful attitude. Seeking peer support or joining online ileostomy patient networks may also bring motivation and inspiration during difficult times.

Integrating Exercise For Wellness

Regular exercise is good for both your physical and emotional health, and it's particularly crucial for ileostomy sufferers. However, it is important to choose activities that are pleasant and appropriate for each individual's fitness level and health status.

Walking, swimming, yoga, and cycling are all great ways to stay healthy without placing too much pressure on your abdomen or ostomy site. It is important to listen to your body and alter intensity or length as required to avoid weariness or pain.

Mental Health & Wellbeing

Coping with an ileostomy may be difficult on mental health, but emphasizing self-care and finding assistance can help manage stress and improve overall well-being. Deep breathing, meditation, and mindfulness are all relaxation strategies that may help you decrease anxiety and build emotional resilience.

Establishing a strong support network of friends, family, healthcare professionals, and other ostomy patients may give vital emotional support and understanding. Furthermore, obtaining professional counseling or therapy might provide ways to deal with the emotional issues of living with an ostomy.

Support Systems For Success

Having a strong support structure in place is critical for ileostomy patients to navigate everyday life and overcome obstacles. This assistance may come from a variety of sources, including family, friends, medical professionals, and internet networks.

Empowering Yourself with Knowledge

Educating yourself on your health, treatment choices, and self-care skills is both empowering and necessary for successfully managing life with an ileostomy.

Use educational materials, support groups, and online forums to keep educated and connected with others experiencing similar issues.

Conclusion

Traveling, socializing, remaining motivated, exercising, prioritizing mental health, establishing support networks, and empowering oneself through information are all important parts of living with an ileostomy. By following these guidelines and tactics, ileostomy patients may live meaningful, active, and confident lives, welcoming new experiences and possibilities with perseverance and optimism.